PREVENTING COLORECTAL CANCER

A Comprehensive Guide to Diagnosis, Treatment, and Beyond.

Stella O. Maurice

GAIN ACCESS TO MORE BOOKS FROM THIS AUTHOR

TABLE OF CONTENTS

INTRODUCTION

"Brooke is the epitome of vigor and health. She exudes grace and happiness. Brooke adores nature. She lives in a remote urban neighborhood which enables her to own a garden. A fifty-two-year-old woman, she devoted her days to taking care of her flourishing garden and taking leisurely walks about her town. For Brooke, the idea of cancer was merely gossip, something that happened to other people but not to her.

Brooke had always taken great satisfaction in her healthy diet and busy lifestyle. She keeps up a lively social circle and is well-known as the town's nutrition expert. Fresh veggies from her garden were plentiful, and she gave them liberally to friends and neighbors.

Life played her card when Brooke began experiencing inexplicable changes in her health. She started to experience ongoing exhaustion, unexplained weight loss, and stomach discomfort. She first thought that these sensations could be caused by stress, aging, or the occasional gastrointestinal ailment. But colorectal cancer was the last thing she thought about, which was understandable given that the disease shared symptoms with other illnesses.

Brooke would have continued self-prediction if not for Sarah, her closest friend who kept nudging her till she agreed to visit the hospital.

The prognosis was unexpected. The unexpected news that Brooke never anticipated hearing when sitting in her doctor's office was, "You have colorectal cancer." Her world was irreparably changed, the room appearing to whirl, and the word "hearsay" taking on new significance.

Her first response was one of incredulity and rage. She had dedicated her life to health and well-being; how could this have happened to her?"

What Is Colorectal Cancer?

The colon and rectum are the two portions that make up the large intestine in the digestive system. The colon, the first portion of the large intestine, is where water and nutrients are absorbed. Solid waste eventually settles in the rectum, the last region, before exiting the body through the anus.

The term "colon cancer" or "colorectal cancer" refers to the uncontrollably and improperly growing cells that line the colon and the rectum. Although this cancer can originate in any of the two parts, most of them start as quiet tumors in the colon. Until these tumors get large, they may grow slowly and show no symptoms.

The rectum or colon can be affected by colon cancer, sometimes referred to as colorectal cancer. It happens when normal cells lining the colon or rectum start to proliferate or alter uncontrolled. They develop into lumps known as tumors as a result. These tumors may initially be harmless. This indicates that while the tumor may grow, it won't move to other colonic regions and probably won't cause any problems. On the other hand, the tumors may develop into malignancies if they are not found and treated quickly.

A tumor is considered malignant once it develops cancer. To make matters more complicated, a malignant tumor has the potential to grow and spread to other parts of the body.

Usually, it takes years for a tumor that is not cancerous to manifest before it turns cancerous. Benign tumors, however, can occasionally turn malignant in a matter of months or years. For this reason, routine screening for colon cancer is crucial.

Collins was no stranger to colorectal cancer's shadow. To him, it wasn't just a life-threatening disease, it was a life-sentence ailment. Having lost his grandfather to colorectal cancer at 64 and his alcohol-loving father at 51, he realized it was time to take control of his health and take on this difficult opponent when he approached his mid-forties.

Collins grew up watching his grandfather languish in pain inflicted on him by colorectal cancer. He also watched his dad struggle because of colorectal cancer. Even though he didn't know much about other extended family members, he knew the colorectal cancerous cell was genetic in his family. Watching his father and grandfather struggle served as a sobering reminder of his possible future as well as a warning tale.

This family history gave Collins the motivation to firmly commit to colorectal cancer screening. He spoke with a genetic counselor, who verified his hereditary tendency. Equipped with this understanding, he commenced routine examinations well ahead of the suggested age, experiencing colonoscopies and genetic testing to enhance the precision of his risk assessment.

Collins was given gloomy news when he obtained the results of one of his examinations. He had a precancerous polyp that might have progressed to malignancy if treatment wasn't received. However, because of his attention to detail, the polyp was removed during the colonoscopy, possibly averting a dire prognosis.

Globally, the incidence of colorectal cancer is rising, yet early detection is believed to boost the chance of a cure. Therefore, early detection is crucial. It is well established that patients with confined cancer tumors, or those whose cancer was detected early, have a greater 5-year survival rate for colorectal cancer cases than do those whose cancer has spread. Specifically, the 5-year survival rate for colorectal cancer in its early stages is 90% or greater, meaning that individuals with this cancer have a very high chance of surviving if they receive an early diagnosis.

Scope Of the Book

Colorectal cancer poses a serious threat to millions of people globally. Nevertheless, there is hope despite the disease's widespread occurrence—hope in the method of prevention. "Preventing Colorectal Cancer" is an informative and comprehensive book that explores the depths of this sneaky illness, providing priceless knowledge and methods to enable people to take charge of their health and lower their risk of colon cancer.

For individuals who wish to comprehend the extent of colorectal cancer and the numerous variables that influence its growth, this book is a goldmine of information. It starts with deciphering the complex nature of colorectal cancer and clearing up any confusion on its underlying causes, hereditary predispositions, and environmental factors. Readers will understand the nuances of the illness through understandable and straightforward language, paving the way for well-informed decision-making.

"Preventing Colorectal Cancer" explores a diversity of preventive procedures, varying from dietary and lifestyle preferences to timely detection strategies and screening initiatives, going beyond simple awareness. It offers doable advice on leading a healthy lifestyle, supported by research, including dietary suggestions, fitness schedules, and stress-reduction techniques.

In addition, the book provides readers with useful tools for self-evaluation, enabling them to recognize their particular risk factors and decide when and how to screen and monitor. It also covers the most recent developments in diagnostic technologies and the significance of routine examinations to identify possible problems early on.

A plethora of information, inspiration, and useful advice can be found in "Preventing Colorectal Cancer," all of which are geared toward lessening the burden of this difficult illness. It serves as a guide for people hoping to make their way through the confusing world of colorectal cancer prevention and toward a healthy, cancer-free future.

CHAPTER 1

Structure Of the Colon and The Rectum

The large intestine includes the colon, the rectum, and the anus. In the last stages of food's passage through your digestive system, it all continues as one long tube that originates in the small intestine.

The gastrointestinal (GI) tract, which is a lengthy, tube-like channel that food goes through in your digestive system, ends with the large intestine. Food waste exits your body through the anal canal, which is where it ends after leaving the small intestine. Food waste is converted into excrement, stored, and eventually excreted in the large intestine, also known as the large bowel. The colon, rectum, and anus arc all part of it. The term "colon" can also refer to the entirety of the large intestine.

Although the large intestine is a single, lengthy tube, various processes occur in different sections of it. The colon, the rectum, and the anus are its three sections. There are more divisions within the colon. The cecum is the entering point, which is roughly six inches long. The ascending colon (which travels up), the transverse colon (which travels across to the left), the descending colon (which travels down), and the sigmoid colon (which heads back across to the right) comprise the remaining segments of the colon.

Individuals have varied mental divisions of the large intestine because there isn't a physical division between the segments. For some, the large intestine is the whole digestive tract minus the anus. The colon, the rectum, and the cecum are also referred to as the three sections of the large intestine. Alternatively, they may refer to it as the colon, although they mean the rectum, the cecum, and the remaining part of the colon.

Function Of the Colon

When the large intestine receives food from the small intestine, the food has passed through the digestive process, liquified, and most of its nutrients have been absorbed. The remaining food must be dehydrated in the colon for it to become stool. It accomplishes this by progressively absorbing electrolytes and water while its muscular system pushes the waste forward. In the meantime, the chemical portion of digestion is finished by bacteria that reside in your colon and feed on the waste to further break it down.

Cecum

A colon's beginning is called the cecum. The ileocecal valve, a tiny tube in the cecum's side, allows the small intestine to feed into it, which is why the cecum's end is truly closed like a pouch. The widest part of the large intestine is located in this pouch, which is the first six inches of the colon. This is the holding area where food enters the large intestine from the small intestine. The colon's muscular contractions start when the cecum fills up.

Colon

Food moves uphill via the transverse colon and finally sideways across the ascending colon. The small intestine is coiled internally and is framed by these segments. The dietary waste that enters the descending colon is primarily solid since any leftover water and electrolytes are absorbed in the ascending and transverse colons. When food waste becomes dry, the colon secretes mucus to bind and lubricate it so that it passes through more easily.

Similar to the small intestine, the big intestine uses periodic muscle contractions to push food forward while simultaneously churning it against its mucous lining. However, the lengthy intestine processes this material at a rate of roughly 24 hours. Here, too, digestion occurs, although not with the help of enzymes as it did in the small intestine. Here, the residual carbs are broken down by beneficial gut bacteria to create essential vitamins (B and K), which are then taken in through the mucosa. It requires more time.

Function Of the Rectum

Rectum

The food waste looks like regular poop by the time it reaches the rectum through the sigmoid colon. Now, the excrement is made up of water, mucus, and indigestible debris that have been discharged from your intestinal mucosa. Approximately 5 ounces of the 16 ounces of liquid food that entered the large intestine would still be in the form of poop. The urge to urinate is triggered when stool enters the rectum. The mass muscular motions of the colon naturally continue in this way.

Anus

The channel through which your excrement will exit your body is called the anus. A muscular sphincter closes it on either side. The internal sphincter on the inside releases waste products automatically. When the time comes, you can release the poop through the control of the outer sphincter. The internal sphincter relaxes in response to nerve signals when feces in the rectum cause the urge to defecate.

The Role of The Colon and Rectum In The Digestive System

In addition to its numerous other roles, the colon is essential for both digestion and waste elimination. The five components of a Colon harden feces, collect nutrients, and water, and transport waste materials toward the rectum.

The majority of the gut's bacteria, which aid in the digestion of substances the body is unable to process on its own, are also found in the colon.

The rectum and colon remove waste from the body, produce and store stool, and collect water and some nutrients from the food and drink we consume.

Food that has partially broken down or processed enters the colon from the small intestine. To pass food through the colon and rectum, certain parts of the colon contract and relax. We refer to this movement as peristalsis.

Food is broken down by microorganisms in the colon into smaller particles. Water and certain nutrients are absorbed by the mucosa's inner layer, known as the epithelium. A semi-solid stool is created from the liquid waste that is still present in the colon.

The mucus produced by the mucosa facilitates the passage of stool via the colon and rectum. More water is taken in from stool as it passes through the colon, making it more solid.

The feces travels from the colon into the rectum. The rectum serves as the stool's holding cavity. The rectum pushes the stool through the anus and out of the body when it is full.

CHAPTER 2

Symptoms And Signs of Colorectal Cancer

While there may be some early warning indicators, colorectal cancer symptoms may be mild or nonexistent in the early stages of the disease. It is possible that colorectal cancer symptoms won't appear until the disease has advanced to stage 2 or higher stages.

The majority of colorectal cancer symptoms are also present in other, less dangerous conditions, such as hemorrhoids, infections, inflammatory bowel syndrome, and irritable bowel syndrome. Because of this, it's simple to write it off as another, less serious illness. Nonetheless, it's crucial to give these symptoms the consideration they require.

Early warning indicators of colorectal cancer in its early stages may include abrupt loss of weight and/or tiny, ribbon-like stool. Other typical early indicators of colorectal cancer consist of the following:

1. Changes in the form, color, and texture of your stool

The form, color, and texture of your stool may noticeably change if you have colon cancer. The stool has a thin, smooth texture and tends to look ribbon-like. It could also seem kind of black.

2. Having trouble passing the stool

Stool passing may also be tough for you, even when you're in the mood to use the restroom. You can also see a change in your bowel habits. These could manifest as bowel incontinence, constipation, constriction of the stools, and incomplete evacuation.

3. Rectal bleeding

Open sores may result from colon cancer, which damages the colon walls. Rectal bleeding follows, which can be minor to severe (and last for extended periods).

4. Blood in stool

One of the most typical indications of colon cancer is rectal bleeding. Blood-stained excrement can occur when the blood and stool combine in the rectum. Additional ailments like hemorrhoids, fissures, Crohn's disease, and bleeding in the digestive tract could also be the cause of this.

5. Mysterious anemia

One of the symptoms of anemia is a low red blood cell count. Oxygen is transported throughout your body by red blood cells. Prolonged and severe rectal bleeding can be a result of colon cancer. Over time, it may cause a considerable loss of blood, which would lead to anemia.

6. Pain in the abdomen or pelvis

One of the first and most prevalent symptoms of colon cancer is abdominal pain. Constant cramping and gas accumulation are possible side effects as well.

7. Losing weight

Toxic compounds released by cancer cells frequently disrupt the digestive tract and alter the process by which food is transformed into energy. This frequently leads to unintended and inexplicable weight loss. It's obvious that something is seriously wrong if, within six months, you unintentionally lose five percent or more of your body weight.

8. Indigestion

One of the typical alterations in bowel motions in colon cancer patients is constipation. A person with colon cancer may experience fewer than three weekly bowel movements.

9. Diarrhea

As opposed to constipation, diarrhea (very loose, regular stool) can also be caused by colon cancer. Certain foods have the potential to exacerbate the condition. Eating meals high in soluble fiber, like oatmeal, white rice, and ripe bananas, is advised in this situation. To replenish lost fluids and avoid dehydration, consume adequate water.

10. Vomiting

Tumors that restrict the bowel and prevent food and waste from passing through can develop as a result of colon cancer. This frequently causes nausea and vomiting, prevents eating, and aids in weight loss.

The initial signs of colon cancer are minor, but they get worse with time. Some of these symptoms don't show up until the cancer has been there for a while. Furthermore, a few of these symptoms are frequent and moderate, making it simple to confuse them for transient pain or discomfort. For instance, a lot of people don't think much about modest stomach aches or notice changes in their stools.

Thankfully, colon cancer is among the most curable (and avoidable) cancer kinds. When detected and treated at a localized stage, the disease has a 91% survival rate. As soon as you observe these or any other colon cancer-related symptoms, you should schedule an appointment with a physician. Therefore, as soon as you notice unusual stomach pain and other signs like blood in your stools, you should give your doctor a call.

Regular cancer screening tests for various disorders, including colon cancer, are also advised. In particular, if there is a family history of colon cancer, routine screening is recommended.

CHAPTER 3

Causes And Risk Factors of Colorectal Cancer

Colorectal cancer arises from mutations in the DNA of colon or rectum cells that may impair their ability to regulate growth and division. These mutant cells frequently perish or come under attack by the immune system. However, certain mutant cells might evade the immune system, proliferate uncontrollably, and develop into a tumor in the rectum or colon.

Although the precise origin of colorectal cancer is unknown, there is solid evidence linking several risk factors to an increased chance of the illness developing. You have some control over the majority of risk variables, but not all of them. The following are a few reasons for colorectal cancer:

Inherited changes in genes

When DNA alterations take place in colon or rectal cells, colon cancer occurs. Certain gene alterations are linked to specific colorectal diseases. Colon cancer is more likely to strike if you inherit genes containing such alterations. The two most prevalent hereditary colorectal cancers are familial adenomatous polyposis

(FAP) and Lynch syndrome. The majority of colorectal cancer cases occur in individuals without a family history of the disease. Nevertheless, up to 1/3 of those who have colorectal cancer have relatives who have already had the disease.

Individuals who have a first-degree relative—a parent, sibling, or child—with a track record of colorectal cancer are more vulnerable. If more than one first-degree relative is impacted or if the relative's cancer diagnosis occurred before the age of 50, the risk is even higher.

In certain instances, the causes of the higher risk are unclear. Due to inherited genes, common environmental conditions, or a mix of these, cancers can "run in the family."

An increased chance of colon cancer is also associated with a family history of adenomatous polyps. Polyps that have the potential to develop into cancer are known as adenomatous polyps. Ask your doctor if you should begin screening for colorectal cancer or adenomatous polyps before the age of 45 if you have a family history of either condition. Telling your close family about any history of adenomatous polyps or colorectal cancer will help them tell their doctors and begin screening at the appropriate age.

Age

While a colon cancer diagnosis can occur at any age, the likelihood increases with age. Although it can strike younger persons, it is far more common after 50. Uncertainty surrounds the rationale behind the rise in colorectal cancer cases among those under 50.

Race and Ethnicity

Your ethnicity and racial background are another uncontrollable risk factor. Non-Hispanic African Americans in the US have the highest risk of developing colorectal cancer and passing away from it. Also, the Ashkenazi Jews, who are Jews of Eastern European heritage, have one of the highest rates of colorectal cancer of any ethnic group worldwide.

History of Polyps or Cancer

You have a larger chance of developing colorectal cancer again if you have had polyps or a prior diagnosis of the disease. You are more likely to get colorectal cancer if you have a history of adenomatous polyps or adenomas. This is particularly true in cases when there are a lot of big polyps or if any of them exhibit dysplasia.

Even if your colorectal cancer was removed, you are still at risk for developing new malignancies in other areas of your colon and rectum. If you had your first case of colorectal cancer when you were younger, your odds of this re-occurring are higher.

Specific Medical Conditions

There is evidence linking certain medical conditions to a higher risk of colorectal cancer. Among them are type 2 diabetes and inflammatory bowel disease (IBD), which includes Crohn's disease and ulcerative colitis. Long-term inflammation of the colon is a symptom of inflammatory bowel disease (IBD). Individuals with long-term IBD, especially those who do not receive treatment, may experience dysplasia. The word "dysplasia" refers to abnormal-looking cells in the colon or rectum that are not cancerous. Over time, they may transform into cancer.

It might be necessary for you to begin screening for colorectal cancer at a younger age and to have screenings more frequently if you have IBD.

Unlike irritable bowel syndrome (IBS), which doesn't seem to raise your risk of colorectal cancer, inflammatory bowel disease (IBD) requires medical attention.

Individuals who have type 2 diabetes, which is typically not insulin-dependent, are more likely to develop colorectal cancer.

Some of the risk factors for type 2 diabetes and colorectal cancer are similar (e.g., being overweight and physically inactive). However, the risk remains elevated for those with type 2 diabetes even after accounting for these variables. Additionally, after diagnosis, their prognosis (outlook) is typically less good.

Diet

Eating a lot of red meat, packaged meats, and diets high in fat increases your risk of colon cancer. When you fry, broil, or grill meat at extremely high temperatures, chemicals are produced that may increase your risk of cancer. The extent to which this may raise your risk of colorectal cancer is unknown.

Low blood levels of vitamin D may also make you more vulnerable. Risk is likely reduced by maintaining a balanced diet that consists primarily of fruits, vegetables, whole grains, and minimal amounts of processed and red meat as well as sugar-filled beverages.

Weight

Your weight is another element that affects diets. Your risk of colorectal cancer rises if you become overweight or obese. Obesity increases the chance of colon and rectal cancer in individuals; however, the association appears to be higher in males. Achieving and maintaining a healthy weight may reduce your risk of colorectal cancer.

Alcohol

Drinking alcohol increases your risk of colorectal cancer whether you drink in moderation or excessive amounts. Moderate to high alcohol intake has been associated with colorectal cancer. Moderate to mild alcohol use has also been linked to some risks. It's advisable to abstain from drinking. If someone does choose to drink, they should only have one drink for women and two for men each day. Numerous health advantages could result from this, including a decreased risk of certain cancer types.

Consuming tobacco

Tobacco usage is one of the main risk factors for cancer. According to American Cancer Research, colon cancer can be directly caused by smoking. Furthermore, 12% of US cases of colorectal cancer share the trait of tobacco use. Long-term tobacco users have a higher risk of developing and dying from colorectal cancer than non-smokers do. In addition to being a prominent cause of lung cancer, smoking is also associated with some other cancers.

Level of activity

Your risk of colon cancer is higher if you do not exercise regularly. Because colon cancer and inactivity are related, making sure you regularly engage in physical activity can significantly lower your risk of colorectal cancer.

Preventive Medication

While it is normal to use drugs for other medical conditions, doing so could put you at risk. For those under the age of 70 who are in good health, this is particularly true when nonsteroidal anti-inflammatory medicines (NSAIDs) are taken over an extended length of time.

Research has indicated that men who survive testicular cancer appear to be more likely to develop colorectal cancer as well as a few other cancers. This could be a result of the therapies they've had, like radiation therapy.

Given that radiation therapy involves some radiation exposure to the rectum, several studies have suggested that men who have undergone radiation therapy for prostate cancer may be at increased risk of developing rectal cancer.

The majority of these studies are based on men who received radiation therapy in the 1980s and 1990s, a time when such procedures were less accurate than they are now. Research is still being done in this area, but it is unclear how more recent radiation techniques affect the risk of rectal cancer.

CHAPTER 4

Types Of Colorectal Cancer

Common Types of Colorectal Cancer

Colorectal cancer can either form in the colon or the rectum. It could be called colon cancer if it originates from the colon. It could be referred to as rectal cancer if it originates in the rectum. Nevertheless, these tumors have a lot in common, regardless of where they originate, which is why they are collectively referred to as colorectal cancer.

Typical forms of colorectal cancer consist of:

1. Adenocarcinoma cancer

Adenocarcinoma is the most prevalent kind of colorectal cancer. Ninety-five percent of instances of colorectal cancer are caused by adenocarcinomas of the colon and rectum. The lining of the colon, or large intestine, the rectum, and the end of the colon are the sites of adenocarcinomas. They frequently begin in the inner lining and move to different layers.

Adenocarcinomas come in two less prevalent subtypes:

- **Mucinous adenocarcinoma:** Mucus makes up around 60% of mucinous adenocarcinomas. Compared to conventional adenocarcinomas, the cancer cells may grow more aggressive and spread more quickly due to the mucus. Ten to fifteen percent of rectal and colon adenocarcinomas are mucinous adenocarcinomas.

- **Signet ring cell adenocarcinoma:** Less than 1% of colon cancer cases are signet ring cell adenocarcinomas. Named for its microscopic look, signet ring cell adenocarcinoma is usually aggressive and may pose greater treatment challenges.

The following are typical symptoms of colorectal adenocarcinoma:

- ★ Pain and discomfort in the abdomen
- ★ Stool containing blood.
- ★ Alterations in digestive patterns, such as constipation or diarrhea
- ★ Thin feces
- ★ Unexpected loss of weight

For colorectal adenocarcinomas, common treatment options include:

★ Chemotherapy

★ Surgery

★ Radiation therapy

★ Targeted therapy

2. Gastrointestinal carcinoid tumors

Neural cells known as neuroendocrine cells, which aid in controlling hormone production, are the site of carcinoid tumor development. These tumors are members of the neuroendocrine tumor (NET) group of cancers. The gastrointestinal system or lungs may become home to slow-growing carcinoid tumor cells. Carcinoid tumors are responsible for half of all small intestinal malignancies and roughly 1% of all colorectal cancers.

Where the tumor grows will determine the possible symptoms. Usually, a carcinoid tumor in the appendix doesn't show symptoms until it starts to obstruct the passageway from the appendix to the intestine, at which point it might cause the fever, nausea, and vomiting associated with appendicitis.

Diverse methods may be used to detect gastrointestinal carcinoid tumors, depending on where they originate. For instance, an appendix tumor may be discovered and removed if it results in appendicitis. During regular screenings, rectal tumors may be found.

Diagnosing carcinoid tumors in the abdominal tract involves several tests, such as endoscopy, colonoscopy, imaging scans, blood tests, and urine testing.

Treatment options for gastrointestinal carcinoid tumors consist of:

- Surgery
- Radiation therapy
- Chemotherapy
- Hormone therapy

Rare Types of Colorectal Cancer

Less than 5% of colorectal cancer cases are caused by other uncommon types of Colorectal cancers.

Primary colorectal lymphomas

This particular kind of colorectal cancer develops in the lymphocyte cells of the lymphatic system. White blood cells called lymphocytes aid the body in the fight against illnesses. Numerous body organs, including the spleen, lymph nodes, bone marrow, thymus, and digestive tract, are susceptible to developing lymphoma. About 5 percent of lymphomas and 0.5 percent of all colorectal tumors are primary colorectal lymphomas. This kind of colorectal cancer is more common in men and typically manifests later in life.

Unexplained weight loss, Indigestion, vomiting, bloating, stomach pain, diarrhea, and other stomach problems are possible symptoms. The diagnosis may require endoscopy and biopsy.

Options for treatment vary but could include:

- Surgery
- Radiation therapy
- Chemotherapy

2. Gastrointestinal Stromal Tumors (GISTs)

Interstitial cells of Cajal (ICCs), a special type of cell present in the lining of the digestive tract, give rise to this uncommon form of colorectal cancer. The stomach is where almost 50% of GISTs form. The rectum is the third most typical site, with the small intestine being the site of most other GIST formations. GISTs are categorized as Sarcomas or tumors that originate in connective tissues, such as deep skin tissues, fat, muscle, blood vessels, bones, nerves, and cartilage.

It usually takes some time for these tumors to enlarge to the point where symptoms appear. On the other hand, they might result in gastrointestinal bleeding. Blood in the vomit or bowel movements may be an indication of the tumor's location. Slow bleeding can eventually result in anemia, a condition that lowers red blood cell counts and produces weakness and exhaustion.

Additional possible symptoms include:

- Stomachache
- Stomach bulge or mass
- Nausea and vomiting
- A low appetite
- Loss of weight
- Swallowing issues

Several imaging tests, a biopsy, a colonoscopy, and an endoscopy are all possible steps in the diagnosis process.

While some smaller GISTs can be addressed with surgery and targeted therapy, others might not require immediate attention.

3. Leiomyosarcoma

Leiomyosarcoma, another type of sarcoma, is essentially defined as "cancer of smooth muscle." Three layers of the leiomyosarcoma-affected muscle type make up the colon and rectum, and they all cooperate to move waste through the digestive system. About 0.1 percent of all cases of colorectal cancer are of this uncommon kind.

Leiomyosarcomas in the colon or rectum may not show any symptoms in the early stages. As the disease spreads, symptoms including exhaustion, weight loss, blood in the vomit, change in feces, and other stomach issues may appear.

 Standard diagnostic procedures, like biopsy, blood tests, and imaging studies, are often used.

Usually, the first step in treatment is surgery to remove the tumor. Chemotherapy and radiation therapy are further therapeutic possibilities.

4.   Melanomas

Skin cancer and melanomas are strongly related. They can originate in any part of the body, such as the colon or rectum, or they can spread from the main melanoma site to the GI tract. Melanomas comprise one to three percent of all gastrointestinal tract malignancies. Since melanomas are incredibly rare, nothing is known about how they form in the colon. A biopsy and further tests may be performed to confirm the diagnosis and establish if the cancer originated in the colon or rectum or spread to other parts of the body.

Treatment options for colorectal melanoma could be:

- ★ Chemotherapy
- ★ Immunotherapy
- ★ Surgery
- ★ Radiation therapy

5. Colorectal Squamous cell carcinoma

Though it is the second most prevalent type of skin cancer, squamous cell carcinomas (SCC) are less common in the colon than they are on the skin. Squamous cells are a specific kind of cell that can be found throughout the body. When these cells begin to grow out of control and develop into cancer, it is known as squamous cell carcinoma. It's unclear why this doesn't happen very often in the colon and rectum.

Colorectal adenocarcinoma-like symptoms, such as stomach problems and changes in stools or bowel habits, may be present. To diagnose this cancer, a colonoscopy is performed along with other tests. It's critical to ascertain whether the cancer originated in the colon or rectum or whether it moved from another part of the body to this area. Although there is no set course of treatment, options include radiation, chemotherapy, and surgery.

Syndromes Associated with Colon Cancer.

If an individual presumes that he/she has an inherited disease linked to colorectal cancer, he/she might consider doing genetic testing. In genetic testing, a sample of the patient's blood, hair, or other bodily fluids is taken and analyzed to check for DNA mutations associated with hereditary syndromes or cancer. Additionally, the patient might be counseled to start screening early and have routine colonoscopies to check for colorectal cancer.

1. Familial Adenomatous Polyposis (FAP)

Approximately 1% of cancers in the colon or rectum are caused by familial adenomatous polyposis (FAP). Colon or rectal polyps numbering in the hundreds or thousands may develop in patients with Familial adenomatous polyposis (FAP).

Since a tumor suppressor gene mutation is most frequently inherited, a parent will typically be impacted. FAP, however, occurs spontaneously in 25% of individuals. Since this gene typically prevents abnormal cell activity, cancerous cells can arise when it is altered.

While polyps can appear in children as young as 10 or 12, they are most frequently discovered in young adults between 20- 40. Colon cancer is a lifetime occurrence for almost all individuals with this disease. Early screening is essential if there is a family history. As a precaution, the doctor might advise colon surgery.

2. Peutz-Jeghers Syndrome (PJS)

This disorder results in the development of a hamartoma, a specific kind of polyp, in the gastrointestinal tract. Mutations in a specific gene (STK11) cause this syndrome, which is inherited from one's parents. It carries a higher chance of developing colorectal cancer in addition to breast, ovarian, and pancreatic cancers. If colon cancer does arise in PJS patients, it typically does so earlier than the usual age of onset.

3. Familial Colorectal Cancer

There are certain individuals whose parents carry genetic disorders that raise their risk of colorectal cancer. Mutations associated with these diseases include those that increase the risk of developing cancer. Lynch syndrome, familial adenomatous polyposis, and other uncommon syndromes are a few examples. Lynch syndrome has been linked to between 2 and 4 percent of colon or rectum cancer cases.

Individuals who have Lynch syndrome are up to 50% more likely to develop colorectal cancer in their lifetime. Lynch syndrome carriers who later develop colorectal cancer typically do so at an earlier age than average.

4. Mutyh-Associated Polyposis (MAP)

MAP is an uncommon, hereditary disorder that results in abnormal tissue growths, or polyps, in various body areas. While most polyps are not cancerous, if left untreated, some can develop into that disease.

MAP frequently results in the growth of several polyps in your colon and rectum. Additionally, polyps can develop in your stomach and small intestine. The risk of colorectal cancer is much higher in those who have this syndrome than in those who do not. When MAP patients are first diagnosed, about half of them also have colorectal cancer. Although some manifest earlier, the majority of these cancers happen between the ages of 40 and 60. Together with other tumors outside of your gastrointestinal (GI) tract, they can also be at risk for duodenal cancer.

If they get early and frequent cancer screenings, many people with MAP can expect to live typical lives. Early detection and removal of polyps is crucial to prevent them from developing into cancer.

5. Cystic Fibrosis (CF)

The hereditary disease known as cystic fibrosis (CF) causes cells in specific organs to produce mucus that is stickier and thicker than usual. Health issues may result from this, particularly with the pancreas and lungs. It's become evident that individuals with cystic fibrosis (CF) are more susceptible to colorectal cancer, which typically manifests at a much younger age than in healthy individuals. This is because improved medical care has made people with CF live longer. Those who have had organ transplants, such as lung transplants, are even more at risk for colorectal cancer. Cystic fibrosis transmembrane conductance regulator, or CFTR, gene mutations are the cause of CF.

Finding families affected by these inherited disorders is crucial because many of them are associated with colon cancer at an early age and are also associated with other cancers. Doctors can prescribe particular actions, including screening and other preventative treatments when the patient is younger when there is early detection.

CHAPTER 5

Diagnostic Tests and Screening Methods

Early diagnosis and treatment make colon cancer manageable. It is recommended by health officials that individuals with an average risk of colorectal cancer start colonoscopy screening at age 45. Patients should talk to their doctors about when to begin screening if they have a family history of the condition, have had benign polyps removed, or have other risk factors including inflammatory bowel disease. Colonoscopy screening may be required for certain individuals as early as age 21. 'At-home tests' are part of the screening process; they evaluate your stool for cancer DNA or blood, which may reveal the presence of precancerous and cancerous colon polyps. Additionally, it consists of three primary exploratory procedures: CT colonographies, sigmoidoscopies, and colonoscopies.

Typically, a sigmoidoscopy is performed every five years, a colonoscopy every ten years, and a stool test every year. Talking to your doctor about the type of test is the best option.

Stool Examination

These examinations examine the stool (feces) for any indications of polyps or colorectal cancer. Many patients find these tests less invasive than others like colonoscopies because they can usually be completed at home. But a higher frequency of these examinations is required. There are three (3) categories for the stool test:

1. The guaiac-based fecal occult blood test (gFOBT): this test looks for blood in the stool by using the chemical guaiac. Your healthcare professional will provide you with a test kit for this examination. Use a brush or stick to get a small amount of stool at home. The stool samples are examined for the presence of blood when you return the test kit to the physician or a laboratory. When choosing gFOBT for colorectal screening, You might be told to abstain from the following before this test because certain foods and medications may alter the results:

i. NSAIDs (non-steroidal anti-inflammatory drugs), such as aspirin, naproxen (Aleve), or ibuprofen (Advil), for seven days before your test scheduled date. (They may induce bleeding, which can result in an incorrectly positive test result.) Note: Before the test, people should try to avoid using NSAIDs for mild pains. However, do not stop taking these medications for this test without first consulting your healthcare physician if you take them regularly for heart issues or other disorders.

ii. Consuming more than 250 mg of vitamin C per day via supplements or citrus fruits and juices three to seven days before testing. (Even if blood is present, this may alter the test's chemicals and provide a negative result.)

iii. Liver, lamb, or other red meats for three days before the test day. (A positive test result could be brought on by blood components in the meat.)

The Guaiac-based Fecal Occult Blood Test is carried out annually.

2. The Fecal Immunochemical Test (FIT): FIT which is approximately 79% accurate in identifying colon cancer, employs antibodies to find blood in the stool. To get started, simply have a bowel movement, gather a little bit of feces, and send it to the laboratory for examination. Everything you need is included in the kit, including a sterile container, a specific envelope for sending, and instructions, and a swab for collecting feces. Most insurance carriers cover FIT, which is easy to use and seamless. It is conducted annually in the same manner as a gFOBT. Patients must repeat FIT every year because polyps may not be bleeding when the test is performed and because the test looks for cancer by looking for blood in the stool. And you still require a colonoscopy even if the results of the FIT test are positive.

3. **The FIT-DNA test:** sometimes called the stool DNA test, combines the results of the FIT with an additional test to look for changed DNA in the feces. To do this test, you must gather a whole bowel movement and send it to a lab where it is examined for blood and changed DNA. This test is taken once every three years.

Flexible Sigmoidoscopy

This examination is used to assess the colon or lower portion of the large intestine. The doctor inserts a short, flexible, illuminated tube into your rectum to do this exam. The doctor can see the interior of the rectum, the sigmoid colon, and the majority of the descending colon thanks to a tiny video camera at the tip of the tube. The doctor examines the lower portion of the colon and the rectum for cancerous growths or polyps. During a flexible sigmoidoscopy examination, tissue samples (biopsies) may be obtained through the scope if necessary. A flexible sigmoidoscopy does not give the physician a full view of the colon. Therefore, flexible sigmoidoscopy by itself is unable to identify cancer or small cell clusters called polyps that may spread farther into the colon and eventually develop into cancer. Sometimes sigmoidoscopy is preferable over colonoscopy because it requires less time to prepare for and conduct the test. Furthermore, anesthetic is frequently not necessary. Compared to colonoscopy, sigmoidoscopy carries a decreased risk of direct injury, such as a rip in the colon or rectum wall (perforation).

Note: A flexible sigmoidoscopy is performed every 5 years, or 10 years if a FIT is performed annually.

Colonoscopy

This is comparable to a flexible sigmoidoscopy, with the exception that the doctor examines the entire colon and the rectum for polyps or cancer using a longer, thinner, flexible tube. Most polyps and certain malignancies can be found and removed by the doctor during the examination. A colonoscopy is also performed as a test of follow-up if an abnormality during one of the other screening procedures is discovered.

Preparing for the colonoscopy

One of the most hated medical procedures on people's to-do lists is the colonoscopy since the unpleasantness of the preparation and test itself is worse than the real one.

Inevitably, for physicians to locate and remove polyps, a clear colon is necessary, and this calls for some planning. The two aspects of colonoscopy preparation are nutrition (diet) and a course of potent laxatives. Although it may seem difficult, following these six steps will make it easy for you:

★ Follow guidelines. Your doctor will give you specific instructions before your exam. These guidelines are meant to assist you in clearing out your digestive tract so that polyps and other anomalies can be easily observed by your doctor, saving you the trouble of having to return for another report. Make sure you comprehend the directions, and contact your doctor if you have any questions.

★ Organize your restroom. Get the liquid laxative that your doctor prescribed, some medicated wipes that include vitamin E and aloe, and a skin-soothing moisturizer (like Vaseline or Aquaphor). To further protect your skin, you might even think about using hemorrhoid cream or diaper rash ointment before prep.

★ Watch what you eat. You must abstain from entire grains, raw fruits and vegetables, nuts, seeds, and meat a few days before the surgery. Rather, your diet will consist primarily of white items, such as cooked or canned fruits and vegetables, along with pasta, bread, and potatoes.

★ Drink clear liquids. You'll follow a clear liquid diet the day before the test; examples include apple juice, Jell-O, clear soft drinks, popsicles, and broth. You can stay hydrated by consuming a lot of liquids. Simply stay away from anything dyed in blue, purple, or red.

★ Make your prep drink better. Many people find it difficult to endure the prep drink. Keep it cold, sip it with a straw, and chew on tart or lemon-flavored candies after every glass to mask the taste to make it more bearable. You can also add powdered drink mix for flavor if the solution isn't already flavored (just make sure it's not red, blue, or purple). Try a lemon. And if you remain uncertain? Consult your physician about the new prep pill; it might be easier for you to take than the prep drink.

★ Follow your schedule. Scheduling the appointment is often the most challenging aspect of a colonoscopy for patients. Aim to keep your screening appointment scheduled, try not to cancel. You'll need to be near a restroom on prep day. You will be sedated on test day, and it will take some time for the drug to take effect.

Colonoscopies are generally well tolerated and safe. The majority of folks can't even recall the steps. It's crucial to monitor your digestive health in between colonoscopies and to let your doctor know if your bowel habits change. Above all, pay attention to rectal bleeding.

Note: Colonoscopies are performed every ten years on individuals without a higher risk of colorectal cancer.

CT Colonography (Virtual Colonoscopy)

A virtual colonoscopy, or computed tomography (CT) colonography, generates images of the entire colon using X-rays and computers. The doctor can examine these images on a computer screen. Although it normally takes thirty minutes, you should plan on spending an hour or more at the hospital.

For this test, your bowel must be empty. This will enable the radiographer to observe your rectum and colon. The day before your test, you must use strong medication (laxatives) to clear your colon. Alternatively, you may need to consume gastrografin, a specific liquid (contrast medium), over the course of one or two days.

Gastrografin is an example of an iodine-containing dye. It aids in improving the clarity of scan images. Additionally, it has laxative properties and may cause diarrhea.

If you take laxatives or gastrografin, you will frequently need to abruptly empty your bowels. It's possible that you're experiencing cramping. After taking gastrografin or the laxatives, it is advisable to remain at home for a few hours so that you are close to a bathroom.

A low-fiber diet may also be necessary for one or two days before to the test.

Drink plenty of clear liquids, such as water, black tea or coffee, squash (without adding red or purple coloring), and clear soup, to avoid being dehydrated.

You might have to quit using iron supplements or other medications that make you constipated. Usually, you give these up a week before the exam.

If you use blood thinners or have diabetes, call the radiology department as soon as you can before your visit. You'll receive more guidelines to adhere to.

Note: A CT scan is performed every five years.

Self-Screening Methods: Know What to Do

Every test has benefits and drawbacks. Discuss with your doctor the benefits and drawbacks of each test as well as the recommended frequency of testing. The following factors primarily determine the best screening technique:

★ Age: The right screening test is chosen based in large part on your age. The majority of guidelines suggest beginning routine tests for colorectal cancer at age 45 or 50. You might have to begin earlier, though, if colorectal cancer runs in your family.

★ Your inclinations: Think about how comfortable you are using various screening techniques. Everyone has benefits and cons. For example, a colonoscopy can be quite successful but can also be painful and need extra preparation. Although non-invasive, FOBT and FIT must be used more regularly. To make an informed choice, talk to your healthcare professional about your preferences and concerns.

★ Your state of health: Your current medical issues and general health may influence which screening test is recommended. Certain examinations, such as colonoscopies, are risky for people with certain medical conditions and demand for anesthesia. Finding the safest and most efficient screening technique requires honest communication about your health state with your healthcare professional.

★ Your individual or family history of colorectal polyps or cancer. In the event that you suffer from a hereditary non-polyposis colorectal cancer (Lynch syndrome) or familial adenomatous polyposis (FAP).

★ The tools at hand for testing and subsequent actions: To find out which screening tests are covered and how often, contact your health insurance provider. This may affect your decision because you may find certain tests to be more affordable. Following a regular screening schedule is crucial, regardless of the screening test you use. In addition to reminding you when your next test is due, your healthcare practitioner can assist you in creating a screening schedule.

A multidisciplinary care team's experience and advice are often needed during the colon cancer treatment process. This group of doctors specializes in treating colon or rectal cancer; however, they have various medical specialties. They collaborate to develop a successful treatment strategy made just for you.

Because colon cancer can be treated with a variety of methods, depending on their area of expertise, numerous doctors may walk you through various treatment options. These physicians may include:

i. Gastroenterologist: This is a Specialist in gastrointestinal and digestive problems.

ii. Surgical oncologist: This is an expert in cancer treatment using surgery.

iii. Colorectal surgeon: This doctor is competent in treating disorders of the colon and rectum.

iv. Radiation oncologists: This doctor specializes in destroying cancer cells with radiation treatment.

v. A Medical oncologist: This doctor focuses on cancer treatments including chemotherapy.

As part of your care team, you may also have meetings with nurses, nutritionists specializing in cancer care, pharmacists, social workers, and psychologists.

Your cancer care team may take into account a number of things while creating and customizing your treatment strategy.

The Importance of Perpetual Colorectal Cancer Screening.

Regular screening can help avoid many colorectal cancers. Precancerous polyps, or abnormal growths in the colon or rectum, can be found by screening and removed before they develop into cancer. Colorectal cancer is very treatable if detected early, which makes screening crucial. Typically, colorectal cancer exhibits no signs in its early stages. It is common for symptoms to emerge when the cancer gets worse.

It is impossible to exaggerate the significance of routine colorectal cancer screening. Regular screening is essential for the following main reasons:

★ Early Detection: In its early stages, colorectal cancer frequently exhibits no symptoms. Frequent screening can find precancerous polyps or cancer in its early stages, when it is most treatable. Treatment results and survival rates can both be considerably increased by early detection.

★ Cancer Prevention: Certain screening procedures, like a colonoscopy, can remove precancerous polyps during the operation in addition to detecting cancer, thereby preventing the development of cancer in the first place.

★ Mortality Reduction: In the US, colorectal cancer ranks as the second most common cause of cancer-related fatalities. Frequent screening lowers mortality rates by detecting cancer at a more curable stage.

★ Reducing Invasive Treatments: When cancer is discovered at an advanced stage, more severe and intrusive therapies including radiation, chemotherapy, and surgery are frequently needed. By detecting cancer at an earlier, more controllable stage, routine screening can help prevent the need for these harsh therapies.

★ Better Quality of Life: People with colorectal cancer may have a higher quality of life as a result of early detection and treatment. It can lessen the mental and physical toll that advanced cancer takes.

★ Cost-Effective: Over time, routine screening for colorectal cancer may prove to be financially advantageous. Early cancer treatment is typically less expensive than late-stage cancer treatment, which frequently necessitates more substantial medical procedures.

★ Customized Risk Evaluation: Screening makes a customized risk evaluation possible. More frequent or earlier tests may be beneficial for people with a family history of colorectal cancer or specific risk factors, as early detection will assist them to manage their individual risk profile.

★ Impact on Public Health: By lowering the total incidence of colorectal cancer, routine screening can have a major positive effect on public health. It can ease the burden on healthcare systems and reduce healthcare expenses.

★ Comfort: Being aware that you are keeping an eye on your health in a proactive manner with routine screenings can ease your mind and lessen the anxiety that comes with worrying about cancer that hasn't been found yet.

★ Encouraging Health Awareness: People who undergo routine screening are more likely to take an active role in their health. It increases knowledge about colorectal cancer and stresses the value of early detection.

CHAPTER 6

Treatment Option for Colorectal Cancer

To determine the full scope of a colon cancer diagnosis, more testing may be required. This is known as the stage of cancer. When developing a treatment strategy, the medical team takes the cancer's stage into account.

Colorectal Cancer Stages

There are four stages of colon cancer: 0 through 4. The lowest figures indicate that all of the cancer is contained within the colon's lining. Stage 4 indicates that the cancer has progressed and expanded to several body parts. Metastatic cancer is the term for cancer that spreads.

The following are included in the colon cancer stage system:

Stage 0: This may be referred to as cancer in situ by medical professionals. When they do, they are referring to abnormal or potentially cancerous cells in the innermost layer of your colon wall, the mucosa.

Stage I: Colorectal cancer in Stage I has penetrated the intestinal wall but hasn't expanded into nearby lymph nodes or past the muscular coat.

Stage II: The cancer has progressed deeper into the intestinal wall but has not reached any neighboring lymph nodes. Stage II colon cancer can be of three types:

Stage IIA: The cancer has penetrated most of the colon wall, but it hasn't reached the outer layer yet.

Stage IIB: Your intestinal wall has been penetrated by cancer, or it has moved into the external layer.

Stage IIC: The cancer has progressed to a nearest organ.

Stage III: Your lymph nodes have been affected by colon cancer at this point. Similar to Stage II colon cancer, Stage III colon cancer is divided into three substages:

Stage IIIA: One to four lymph nodes have been affected by cancer that started in the first or second layers of your colon wall.

Stage IIIB: Only one to three lymph nodes are affected, but additional layers of your colon wall are affected by the cancer. Stage IIIB colon cancer also refers to cancer that has progressed to four or more lymph nodes but affects fewer layers of the colon wall.

Stage IIIC: Four or more lymph nodes and the outermost layer of your colon are affected by cancer. Stage IIIC colon cancer also includes cancer that has metastasized to one or more lymph nodes and a nearby organ.

Stage IV: The cancer has metastasized, or spread, to different parts of the body, such as the ovaries, liver or the lungs:

Stage IVA: This is the stage when the cancer has progressed to a single organ or to lymph nodes located a greater distance from the colon.

Stage IVB: More lymph nodes and more than one far away organ have been affected by the cancer.

Stage IVC: Abdominal tissue, lymph nodes, and distant organs are affected by cancer.

Colorectal Cancer Treatment

Surgery is typically required as part of colon cancer treatment to remove the cancerous tumor. The location and stage of the cancer will determine your treatment options. When developing a treatment plan, your medical staff also takes into account your general health and your choices. You must carefully consider all of your options and balance their advantages with any possible disadvantages or risks. You will learn more about the many colon cancer treatment options in this book, along with what to anticipate from each, enabling you to make an informed choice with your doctor about which is most suitable for you. They may utilize one treatment after another or in combination. Various approaches to treating colon cancer include:

A. Surgery

When treating early-stage colon cancer, surgery is usually the first step. The kind of surgery you will undergo depends on the stage of your cancer, the location of the cancer in your colon, and the intended outcome of the procedure.

There are two types of colon cancer surgery:

i. **Local excision and polypectomy:** During a colonoscopy, most polyps and some stage 0 and stage I tumors (early colon cancerous cells) can be removed. During a colonoscopy, the surgeon uses a colonoscope, which is a long, flexible tube with a video camera attached to the end. The surgeon gently pushes it into your colon after inserting it into your rectum. During a colonoscopy, the surgeon can carry out both a local excision and a polypectomy.

During a polypectomy, the surgeon makes a base incision and removes the cancerous parts of the polyp (which resembles a mushroom stem).

A little more work goes into a local excision procedure. The surgeon removes a tiny quantity of healthy tissue from the colon wall and tiny cancerous cells on the inside lining of your colon using instruments seen through a colonoscope.

ii. **Colectomy:** During a colectomy, your colon may be removed entirely or in part by the surgeon. Additionally, they will remove nearby lymph nodes.

There are two ways a surgeon can carry out a colectomy:

a. An open colectomy involves making a single, lengthy incision across the abdomen to execute the procedure.

b. Laparoscopic-assisted colectomy: In this procedure, multiple tiny incisions are made while using specific instruments to complete the surgery. They make use of a laparoscope, which is a long, thin, lighted tube with a tiny camera and an attached light at the end. This gives the surgeon access to see the inside of your abdomen.

Possible Adverse Effects of Colorectal Cancer Surgery

Pain and soreness where the surgeon made the incision are typically the side effects of colon cancer surgery.

Constipation or diarrhea following surgery are also possible side effects, however these usually go away with time. You're may feel itchy in the area surrounding your stomach if you have a colostomy, the irritation is caused by the incision the surgeon made in your abdominal wall.

A lot of people need to retrain their bowels after surgery. It could take some time and help to complete this. In case your bowel function is not properly controlled, you should speak with your physician.

B. Palliative Care

Palliative care is a specialized medical field that addresses the management of pain and other symptoms associated with life-threatening illnesses. An interdisciplinary team of medical specialists provides palliative care. Physicians, nurses, and other people with specialized training may be part of the team. Enhancing the lives of those suffering from severe illnesses and their families is their main objective.

Palliative care is an additional safety net for patients receiving cancer therapy. Palliative care is frequently given in addition to any curative or additional therapies you may be undergoing. Palliative care can help cancer patients feel better and survive longer when combined with all other approved treatments.

C. Immunotherapy

Immunotherapy is a pharmacological treatment which uses your immune system to combat cancer. Since cancer cells hide from the immune system to live, your body's disease-fighting immune system may not target cancer. Your immune system is blinded by cancer cells and is unable to identify them. Immunotherapy obstructs this process. It aids the cells of the immune system in locating and eliminating cancerous cells.

Usually, immunotherapy is only used in cases with advanced colon cancer. Your doctor might run tests on your cancer cells to see how likely it is that they will react to this treatment.

If certain gene changes are detected in your colon cancer cells, the doctor may recommend medications called checkpoint inhibitors. These may include an elevated amount of microsatellite instability (MSI-H) or alterations in one of your mismatch repair (MMR) genes. If surgery is not able to eliminate your cancer, if it has metastasized—spread to other parts of your body—or if it has returned after therapy (recurrent cancer), the doctor may use these medications to treat you.

Possible Adverse Reactions to Immunotherapy

Immunotherapy medication side effects could include:

- ➤ nausea
- ➤ Appetite loss
- ➤ exhaustion
- ➤ Constipation
- ➤ Cough
- ➤ Itchiness/Irritation
- ➤ Joint discomfort

Less frequently, more serious side effects including skin irritation occur. While receiving treatment, some people may have autoimmune reactions or infusion reactions.

D. Chemotherapy

Chemotherapy is a medical procedure that involves injecting or taking anti-cancer drugs intravenously. Most areas of your body can receive these drugs since they enter your bloodstream and move throughout it.

Chemotherapy is a common treatment for colorectal cancer. Stages II, III, and IV are where it's frequently used. Still, there is disagreement among specialists over the appropriate use of chemotherapy for stage II colorectal tumors.

The surgeon may suggest adjuvant chemotherapy (chemotherapy after surgery) if there are particular circumstances that increase the chance of cancer returning.

During the course of treating your colon cancer, your doctor may administer chemotherapy at various intervals. For instance, they could administer:

★ **Adjuvant chemotherapy:** Adjuvant chemotherapy is used after surgery with the intention of eliminating any cancer cells that may have been missed by the surgeon during the surgery because they were too small to view. Also, it is used to eradicate cancer cells that might have migrated from the underlying colon (or rectal) cancer and become embedded in other body areas that are too small for the medical professional to detect using imaging tests. Adjuvant chemotherapy will reduce the likelihood of cancer returning.

★ **Neoadjuvant chemotherapy prior to surgery:** This treatment aims to reduce the size of your cancer so that it can be more easily removed. It may also be used with radiation. Usually, rectal cancer is treated in this manner.

When advanced cancer has spread to other organs, such as the liver, chemotherapy might be used to treat it.

Chemotherapy aids in tumor shrinkage, relieving whatever problems they may be inflicting. Chemotherapy may prolong your life and improve your quality of life, but it won't always be a cure for cancer.

Before surgery, chemotherapy may also be used to reduce a large tumor so that it is easier to remove.

Chemotherapy can also be used to treat colon cancer symptoms that cannot be treated surgically or have migrated to other parts of the body.

Possible Adverse Reactions to Chemotherapy

Potential adverse effects of chemotherapy vary depending on the kind and amount of the treatment. Additionally, it will depend on how long you receive it.

Typical adverse effects of chemotherapy may include:

- vomiting and queasiness
- loss of hair
- Diarrhea
- Appetite loss or weight loss
- Changes in Skin
- Changes in nails

- mouth blisters/sores
- The red blood cells in your bone marrow may potentially be affected by chemotherapy.

The majority of chemotherapy side effects disappear gradually after your treatment is over. Chemotherapy is administered by doctors in cycles, with a rest interval in between to allow the patient's body to adjust to the side effects. Cycles typically last two or three weeks, but the schedule will change based on the drugs you're taking.

E. Radiation Therapy

Radiation therapy uses powerful radiation beams to focus on cancer cells. Protons, X-rays, and other sources are possible sources of the energy. Given that this kind of tumor usually returns close to its original site, it is frequently utilized to treat rectal cancer. Radiation therapy is not a frequently used treatment for colon cancer by medical professionals.

Before surgery, radiation treatment can help a large cancer shrink so that it is easier to remove. Radiation therapy may be used to treat symptoms like discomfort when surgery is not an option. Some patients receive chemotherapy and radiation therapy concurrently. Possible adverse reactions to radiation therapy

The following are potential side effects of radiation therapy:

- Difficult wound recovery if you have radiation therapy prior to surgery.
- Skin irritation (which could manifest as redness, peeling, or blistering) at the radiation beam target region.
- Nausea
- Exhaustion/fatigue
- The symptoms of rectal irritation include painful bowel motions, diarrhea, and blood in the stool.
- Bladder irritation may result in symptoms like burning while urinating, blood in your urine, or the desire to use the restroom more frequently.
- Bowel incontinence or leaking of stool.
- Adhesions, scarring, and fibrosis, which cause the tissues in the treated area to stay together.
- Sexual problems (women's vaginal discomfort, men's erection problems)

When treatment is over, the majority of radiation therapy side effects should fade away, but some may persist. Consult your doctor right away if you experience any persistent side effects so they can help you manage or lessen them.

F. Medication with Specificity

Targeted drug therapy makes use of medications that target specific compounds found in cancerous cells. Cancer cells can be killed by specific medication therapies that block these substances. Chemotherapy is usually given in addition to targeted medications. Usually, they are only given to patients with advanced colon cancer.

Possible Adverse Consequences

Depending on the kind you receive, targeted medication therapy may have different adverse effects. Possible side effects include:

- tiredness
- bleeding
- loss of appetite
- Weariness or excessive fatigue
- Vomiting
- Mouth sores/blisters
- Migraines
- high blood pressure
- Low levels of white blood cells (may raise the risk of infections)
- Tiredness

A few things, such as your general health and any previous treatments you've had, will determine which regimen you should utilize. The doctor will try a different regimen if the first one doesn't work.

G. Embolization and Ablation

When stage IV colon cancer has spread to multiple tiny tumors in the liver or lungs, the surgeon may choose to remove the tumors surgically or use alternative methods, such as embolization or ablation, to kill them.

Once the surgeon has surgically removed all of the major cancer in your colon (or rectum), they may employ ablation or embolization to eradicate minor cancerous cells in other areas of your body.

Possible adverse reactions to ablation

There are many different kinds of ablation methods. When a tumor is less than 4 cm across, doctors employ ablation procedures to eliminate it instead of surgically removing it.

The following are possible ablation therapy adverse effects:

- High temperature/fever
- Stomachache
- Unusual liver test

- Liver disease/infection

- Bleeding in the chest cavity or abdomen

Though they are uncommon, severe problems can happen.

Embolization

When treating liver tumors, the doctor employs embolization. To lessen or stop the blood supply to the tumor, they will inject a drug directly into an artery in your liver during this process.

The following are possible embolization adverse effects:

- Fever

- Nausea

- Stomachache

- Inflammation of the gallbladder

- liver disease/ infection

- Unusual liver test

- Clots in the main blood arteries of your liver

Patients don't usually have to stay in the hospital to receive embolization or ablation procedures.

Clinical Trials

Since every person is unique, their response to therapy for colorectal cancer will also be unique. As long as you receive timely and accurate therapy, you can be optimistic about the future.

While most colon cancer patients experience no recurrence, approximately 35 to 40 percent of patients who undergo surgery, either with or without chemotherapy, may experience a recurrence of the cancer within three to five years after treatment.

Standardized, Routine Therapies May Not Always Work.

Nonetheless, experimental therapy hold potential. Clinical trials are used by researchers to constantly test new therapeutic approaches. Usually, those who are not participating in the trial cannot access them. Many people are optimistic and believe that experimental treatments are worthwhile even though there are no guarantees they will be helpful.

Researchers and medical professionals are constantly searching for more effective strategies to manage colorectal cancer and its patients. In order to improve science, scientists and health care professionals design research studies (also known as clinical trials) using volunteers. All FDA-approved medications have undergone clinical trial testing.

All stages and varieties of colorectal cancer are treated via clinical trials. Modern colon cancer treatments are the subject of numerous trials aimed at determining their safety, efficacy, and potential superiority over existing treatments. Some concentrate on enhancing current therapies.

Clinical trials assess new medications, new therapeutic regimens, new approaches to radiation or surgery, and new combinations of treatments.

CHAPTER 7

Coping With a Colorectal Cancer Diagnosis/ Treatment

Any cancer treatment may have unintended consequences or alter your physical and emotional state. Even while receiving the same treatment for the same type of cancer, people might not encounter the same side effects for a variety of reasons. Because of this, it may be difficult to gauge how you will feel during therapy.

It's common to worry about side effects when you are ready to begin cancer therapy. That being said, it is comforting to know that your medical team will make every effort to minimize and avoid adverse effects. Palliative care, also known as supportive care, is a component of cancer treatment. Regardless of your age or the stage of your disease, it is a crucial component of your treatment approach.

Handling Therapeutic Side Effects

The stage of the cancer, the duration and dosage of treatment, and your overall health are some of the variables that will affect your physical health.

During their treatment for colorectal cancer, many patients experience dietary difficulties (eating inability).

Discuss what you are experiencing with your medical staff on a regular basis. Notifying them of any new adverse effects or modifications to current side effects is crucial. They can find ways to manage or relieve your side effects to help you feel more relaxed and possibly prevent any side effects from getting worse if they are aware of how you are feeling.

Maintaining a record of your side effects could be beneficial in order to facilitate discussions about any adjustments with your medical team. Treatment for cancer is known to have serious negative effects. Chemotherapy, for instance, can result in decreased blood counts, nausea, and even vomiting in addition to hair loss. Some medications produce tingling or pain in the nerves, while some cause rashes. Patients may have varying experiences and varied side effects from various cancer treatments. It is crucial that patients and doctors have regular conversations about a patient's particular symptoms so that the treatment plan can be modified to help the patient feel better.

After therapy is finished, adverse effects might occasionally persist. Doctors refer to this as chronic side effects. Late effects are side effects that manifest months or years after the start of treatment.

One of the most crucial aspects of survivorship care is managing late effects and long-term ones.

Handling the Social and Emotional Fallout of Colorectal Cancer Diagnosis

Receiving a cancer diagnosis can have social and emotional repercussions. This could entail controlling your stress level or coping with a range of emotions, including anger, worry, and grief. People sometimes have a hard time telling their loved ones how they really feel sometimes. Certain people have discovered that speaking with a counselor or oncology social worker can help them come up with better coping mechanisms and conversation starters around cancer.

Methods like yoga, mindfulness, and meditation can help reduce stress and enhance emotional health. You can include these techniques into your everyday routine to help you relax.

Throughout treatment, you can enhance your general well-being and increase your energy levels by following your healthcare team's recommendations for eating a nutritious diet and doing frequent exercise.

It's normal to want to retreat, but make an effort to stay in touch with others. Engaging in enjoyable activities and engaging with loved ones can have a positive emotional impact.

Recognize that living with colorectal cancer is an ongoing process. Establish reasonable objectives for yourself and acknowledge minor victories along the way. Pay attention to what you can manage and adjust when circumstances change.

Living as a Colorectal Cancer Survivor

Treatment for colorectal cancer can eradicate the disease in many cases. Treatment completion can be thrilling and worrisome at the same time. Even though you're happy that your treatment is over, it might be difficult to stop worrying that the cancer will return. Having cancer is a common cause of this.

Some individuals may never fully recover from colorectal cancer. In an effort to keep the cancer under control for as long as possible, some patients may get regular chemotherapy, radiation therapy, or other treatments. It can be challenging and extremely frustrating to figure out how to live with cancer that does not get better.

Plan for Survivorship Care

Discuss creating a plan for your survivorship care with your doctor. This strategy may consist of:

- A recommended itinerary for additional examinations and tests

- a list of potential long-term or late-term side effects from your medication, along with warning signs and when to call your doctor.

- A schedule of additional examinations that you may require in the future, like screening tests for cancers other than breast cancer or early detection tests.

- Advice on how to make adjustments to your diet and physical exercise that may help you feel better and potentially reduce the likelihood that the cancer will return

- Reminders to schedule regular check-ups with your primary care physician (PCP), who will oversee all aspects of your general health care, consisting of any necessary cancer screenings.

Post-Colorectal Cancer Follow-Up

Following the completion of your treatment, you will probably see your doctor for years to come. Going to your follow-up appointments is significant. Your doctors will inquire about any issues you may be having at these appointments, and they may perform examinations, lab tests, or imaging tests to check for side effects from therapy or symptoms of cancer returning.

The stage of your tumor and the likelihood that it will return will influence how frequently you need to have testing and follow-up appointments.

There may be adverse consequences from almost any cancer treatment. While some could pass after a few days or weeks, others might linger for a very lengthy period. It's possible for some adverse effects to manifest years after treatment is completed. You should discuss any changes, issues, or worries you have with your doctor during your appointments, as well as any questions you may have.

Doctor Visits and Tests

Many doctors will advise you to undergo a physical examination and some of the tests indicated below every three to six months during the first few years following your surgery, and then about every six months for the following few years, if there are no lingering symptoms of cancer. This may be less common in those who have received treatment for early-stage cancers.

Colonoscopy

Generally speaking, your doctor will advise a colonoscopy for you to have approximately a year following surgery. The majority of people won't require another one for three years if outcomes are healthy. Future exams can often be scheduled approximately every five years if the exam results are normal. The test may need to be performed more frequently if the colonoscopy reveals abnormal regions or polyps.

Protoscopy

In the event that your rectal cancer was removed via transanal excision (via your anus), your doctor will probably advise having a proctoscopy approximately every three to six months for the first few years after surgery, and then every six months or so for the following few years. This enables the doctor to closely examine the region where the cancer was in order to determine whether the cancer may be relapsing.

Imaging Examinations

The stage of your cancer in addition to variables will determine the likelihood that your doctor suggests imaging testing. For people with a greater chance of recurrence, particularly in the early years following treatment, CT scans may be performed on a frequent basis, such as once every six months to a year. For the first several years following the removal of liver or lung tumors, patients may undergo scans every three to six months.

Blood Test for Tumor Markers

A chemical known as a tumor marker called carcinoembryonic antigen (CEA) is present in the blood of certain patients with colorectal cancer. Before starting treatment, doctors use a blood test to measure this marker's levels.

At your follow-up appointment, which is usually scheduled every 3 to 6 months for the first few years following treatment and then every 6 months or so for the next few years, it can be examined again if it was high initially and then went down to normal after surgery. If the CEA level increases once more, it may indicate that the cancer has returned. To determine the location of the recurrence, imaging tests or colonoscopies may be performed.

Tumor marker levels are unlikely to be useful as a predictor of recurrence if they were not raised at the time the cancer was first discovered.

CHAPTER 8

Prevention of Colorectal Cancer and Lifestyle Modifications

Starting at age 45, frequent colorectal cancer screenings are the most effective method to lower your chance of developing the disease.

The majority of colorectal tumors start out as abnormal growths called precancerous polyps in the colon or rectum. Years may pass before an invasive cancer form in the colon due to the presence of such polyps. In the early stages, they might not even show any symptoms.

Precancerous polyps can be identified by colorectal cancer screening and removed before they develop into cancer. Colorectal cancer is avoided in this way. Moreover, screening can detect colorectal cancer early on, when therapy is most effective.

Additional strategies to avoid colorectal cancer include:

A. Diet

> ➤ **Limit your consumption of red and processed meat:** Studies have shown that the risk of colorectal cancer rises

by 18% for every two slices (50 grams) of processed lunchmeat consumed daily. Consuming red meat raises the risk of colorectal cancer by 12% for every 100 grams. For this reason, it's so much better to substitute meals with chicken, fish, and beans for red and processed meat.

➢ **Consume healthy diets:** consume a range of fruits, vegetables, and whole grains as part of a nutritious diet. Minerals, Fiber, Vitamins and antioxidants found in fruits, vegetables, and whole grains may help prevent cancer. Consuming a diet consisting in fruits, vegetables, and whole grains is very helpful in preventing cancer. This is a result of their high fiber, vitamin, mineral, and antioxidant content.

Pick a choice of fruits and vegetables to ensure you are getting a variety of minerals and vitamins.

➢ **Increased fiber consumption:** consumption of fiber should be increased because research has revealed that fiber consumption considerably lowers the risk for some kinds of colon cancer. Studies have indicated that an increase of five grams of fiber consumed daily can cut the mortality rate from colon cancer by 18%.

➢ **Recognize your fats:** The foods we eat include both "good" and "bad" fats. Colon cancer may be prevented in part by omega-3 polyunsaturated fats, which are found in nuts, seeds, and a variety of seafood. They reduce colon cancer cells by lowering inflammation and favorably affecting hormone signaling. Extensive randomized controlled studies are being conducted to ascertain the precise impact and necessary dosage.

Additionally, maintaining a healthy body weight lowers your chance of colon cancer, which is another benefit of omega-3s.

Conversely, there may be a positive correlation between saturated fat and the occurrence of colon cancer. dishes like butter, ice cream, red meat, and fried dishes include these fats.

> **Consider vitamin D:** Inadequate levels of this vitamin are prevalent in the US and have been connected to a rise in the incidence of colon cancer. You may maintain your levels within a healthy range by getting some sunshine each day and consuming foods high in vitamin D, such as eggs, salmon, and plant-based milk fortified with vitamin D.

For people between the ages of 1 and 70, 600 IU of vitamin D should be taken daily: for infants under the age of one, 400 IU, and for individuals above the age of 70, 800 IU.

B. Healthy Decisions

According to certain research, persons can lower their chance of getting colorectal cancer by doing the following:

> **Engaging or increasing physical activity:** Make an effort to exercise for at least half an hour most days. If you haven't exercised, begin cautiously and increase to 30 minutes over time.
>
> You can reduce your risk of colon cancer by up to 25% by integrating daily walks, gardening, gym sessions, or other forms of exercise in your regimen. People who regularly exercise also have a lower chance of dying after receiving a diagnosis.
>
> Additionally, consult a medical expert prior to beginning an exercise regimen.

> **Maintaining a healthy weight:** It's critical to retain an appropriate physique because obesity increases the risk of colon cancer. If your weight is within a healthy range, try to keep it there by eating well and exercising every day. Start an exercise regimen if you are overweight in order to lose weight and control your caloric intake.
>
> Inquire with your medical staff about safe approaches to accomplish your objective. Reduce your calorie intake and increase your physical activity to gradually lose weight.

➢ **Restricting alcohol consumption:** Research analysis showed that high versus low alcohol drinking elevated the risk of colon cancer by 15%. Alcohol destroys cells, alters hormone responses, and interferes with the absorption of nutrients and weight. The best course of action is to either abstain from alcohol completely or, if you must, to limit your intake to no more than one drink for women and two for men every day.

➢ **Avoid or Quit smoking:** Smoking appears to have the strongest correlation with colon cancer of all the factors of the illness. It's also the action that raises the risk to the greatest degree. Compared to nonsmokers, smokers have a 50% increased risk of colon cancer.

The only method for smokers to lower their vulnerability to risk is to give up completely. It could be difficult, so think about discussing medication or counseling with your doctor.

Dietary Suggestions to Prevent Colorectal Cancer.

Your diet and beverages can be effective preventative measures against colorectal cancer. Your Gut health is a major factor in colon and rectal health, and it can be enhanced with a regular, nutrient-rich diet.

Consider food as medicine; by choosing your foods wisely, you may provide your body system with the nutrition it needs to either prevent or combat cancerous cells. Some foods to include in your diets are:

Captivating fruits: Fruits are a great source of fiber, antioxidants, and phytochemicals, all of which lower the risk of colon cancer and other digestive problems. Fruits including apples, cranberries, blueberries, cantaloupes, mangoes, oranges, grapefruit, cherries, red cabbage, and pears are some delectable and healthful options.

Nuts: Rich sources of fiber, antioxidants, and healthful fatty acids, nuts help lower the risk of colon cancer and type 2 diabetes. Tree nuts—almonds, cashews, hazelnuts, pecans, pistachios, flaxseed, walnut, and macadamia nuts—are the greatest options.

Non-starchy vegetables: A variety of vegetables are rich in fiber, vitamins, minerals, and phytochemicals that improve health. On the other hand, consuming too many starchy vegetables, like potatoes, corn, and peas, can raise your chance of type 2 diabetes, a dangerous condition that also raises your risk of colon cancer. As a result, it's advisable to concentrate on non-starchy veggies including kale, bok choy, legumes, tomatoes, lettuce, spinach, celery, cucumbers, broccoli, cabbage, brussel sprouts, edamame, carrots, and cauliflower.

Legumes and beans: Legumes and beans, such as soybeans, lentils, black beans, red beans, garbanzo beans/chick peas, kidney beans, and pinto beans, are a great source of protein, fiber, and vitamins B and E. Legumes and beans not only lower the risk of colon cancer but also lower blood sugar and cholesterol.

Fresh fish: A diet rich in omega-3 fatty acids can help lower inflammation throughout the body. Examples of these fish are herring, mackerel, salmon, sardines, and tuna. This is significant because ongoing inflammation has been connected to numerous cancers, including colon cancer, by causing constant cell turnover.

White meat: Growth of tissues and the development of muscles depend on an adequate supply of protein. But there is clear evidence linking red and processed meats—like pepperoni, hot dogs, lamb, and cold cuts—to a higher risk of colon cancer. White meats, including lean/skinless chicken and turkey, tofu, and eggs are healthier substitutes.

Complete grains: Whole grains go well with fresh fish, white meats, and eggs since they are full of fiber. Brown rice, tortillas, oatmeal, quinoa, and barley are the healthiest choices.

Diary: Try options that are lower in saturated fats such as skim milk, low fat cheese and diary alternatives (soy based foods and nut milks).

Beverages: select beverages that has no added sugar such as water, green tea, coffee and white tea.

Colorectal Cancer Prevention for People with A High Risk.

Certain medications may lower the chance of colon cancer or polyps. For example, there is evidence that frequent usage of aspirin or aspirin-like medications reduces the incidence of polyps and colon cancer. However, it's unclear how much and for how long would be required to lower the risk of colon cancer. Daily aspirin use carries certain hazards, such as bleeding in the digestive tract and ulcers.

These choices are typically limited to those who have a high risk of developing colon cancer. Insufficient evidence supports the recommendation of these medications for those with an average risk of colon cancer.

Talk to your medical team about your risk factors if you have a higher-than-average risk of colon cancer to see whether taking preventive medication is safe for you.

Aromatic Blends to Prevent Colorectal Cancer

Studies indicate that the phytochemicals present in spices such as cinnamon, ginger, garlic, turmeric, and allspice may have anti-cancer properties. When cooking, add these spices to your food to make it healthier. Remember that a pinch or a teaspoon of spices has the power to completely change a dish. The spices include:

Tumeric: Curcumin, the ingredient that gives turmeric its yellow color, is responsible for making it one of the spices with the most researched anti-cancer properties. Studies conducted in vitro (in test tubes) suggest that curcumin may have chemopreventive properties. While it can interact with many chemotherapy medications and raise the risk of bleeding due to its antiplatelet qualities, there is some preliminary evidence that it may have some clinical use in certain individuals with head and neck cancers, prostate cancer, or gastrointestinal cancers. This mildly flavored spice is commonly used in blends for Indian curries. Additionally, it pairs nicely with rice dishes, veggies, and eggs.

Garlic: Garlic has several phytoconstituents, but some have potent anti-cancer properties, such as SAC, allicin, DAS, SAMC, DATS, and DADS.

Because of their numerous targets and low toxicity, a few active metabolites of garlic have been shown to be crucial in the death of cancerous cells. Studies have shown that consuming large amounts of garlic may lower the incidence of colorectal cancer, probably because of chemicals that include sulfur. Crush or chop fresh garlic and let it aside to generate allicin for five to ten minutes before cooking. The flavor of beans, vegetables, meats, stews, and sauces is enhanced with a small amount of garlic.

Ginger: When used as a cancer treatment, ginger is thought to be 10,000 times more potent than chemotherapy. It is a naturally occurring antioxidant that fights cancer. In addition to aiding in the killing of cancer cells, the active ingredients 6-gingerol and 6-shogaol have anti-cancer qualities against the gastrointestinal tract. A variety of potent substances, such as gingerol, are found in ginger root. Gingerols change into other substances with anti-inflammatory and antioxidant properties when heated or dried. Ginger has a strong aroma and tastes great in baked products, tea, soups, and stir-fries.

Allspice: The dried berries of a South American tree are the source of allspice. Contrary to its name, this isn't a spice blend. Allspice contains a wealth of phytochemicals, phenolic acid, and flavonoids. Research indicates that high concentrations of allspice may aid in preventing the growth of cancer. Allspice earned its name because it tastes like a mixture of nutmeg, cloves, and cinnamon.

Cinnamon: The dried bark of trees is the source of cinnamon. It comes in powdered form or as sticks of curled bark. Studies in the lab have concentrated on the anticancer effects of its main ingredient, cinnamaldehyde. This adaptable spice, which is most frequently used in baking, tastes well in both savory and sweet recipes. The potential benefits of cinnamon for treating and preventing cancer have been extensively researched. Overall, the research indicating that cinnamon extracts may prevent cancer is restricted to experiments conducted on animals and in test tubes. Try adding flavor to stews or drinks with the cinnamon sticks. The powdered version enhances taste.

CHAPTER 9

Cancer and Stress

The diagnosis of cancer, the treatment and the survivorship can be extremely exhausting. It has been demonstrated that stress influences the formation, spread, and metastasis of tumors. The immune system is a primary facilitator in the relationship between stress and the development of cancer, even if other immune-independent systems also have a significant impact in this regard.

The biological stress response, which includes the release of substances in the circulatory system and locally within central and peripheral tissues, is how a stressor might impact the brain event body. Studies have indicated that stress might have an adverse effect on general health problems. Stress can lead to mental health issues and have an impact on the adoption of harmful behaviors.

Research indicates that individuals with long-term stress are frequently more prone to exhibit symptoms of anxiety, depression, binge or overeat, and lead unproductive lives. Prolonged stress can even lead to bodily symptoms including weariness, headaches, and insomnia. Not only is that potentially harmful, but new research also indicates that stress may contribute to the development of cancer. Chronic stress, also known as long-term stress, can alter the body physically. Chronic stress could affect a tumor's ability to grow and spread, even though it hasn't been shown to raise the risk of cancer. The release of norepinephrine is probably partially to blame for this. One hormone connected to stress is norepinephrine.

Stress Reduction Strategies

Stress relief can be achieved through nearly any type of physical exercise. Exercise is a great way to decompress, even if you're not athletic or in high physical condition.

Your feel-good endorphins and other naturally occurring brain chemicals that improve your sense of well-being can be increased by physical activity. Refocusing your mind on your body's activities is another benefit of exercise. With this renewed concentration, your mood can improve and your daily annoyances can fade. So get moving and do anything like go for a walk, jog, work in your garden, clean your home, ride a bike, swim, lift weights, or do the vacuum.

1. Look for a humorous angle.

Just as physical activities release endorphins, laughter also does so, according to research. A good sense of humor is not a cure-all for all problems. Even if you have to fake a laugh through your grumpiness, it can make you feel better. Laughing helps to relieve mental exhaustion. Positive physical changes in the body are also induced by it. Laughing causes your stress reaction to flare up and then subside. When it comes to stress relief, hanging out with one's goofiest pals or losing yourself on YouTube can be helpful. Thus, enjoy some lighthearted reading or telling, comic viewing, or time spent with your humorous pals.

2. Practice Meditation

You quiet the chaotic flow of thoughts that might be overflowing your head and giving you stress during meditation. A state of balance, tranquility, and quiet that you can achieve via meditation can benefit your general health as well as your mental health. We can improve our well-being through meditation.

Anywhere, at any time, you can engage in guided meditation, guided imagery, mindfulness, visualization, and other types of meditation. You may meditate, for instance, while taking a stroll, taking the bus to work, or while you're waiting at the doctor's office. You can practice deep breathing anyplace, too.

3. Interact with other people.

It could be a good idea for you to isolate yourself when you're upset and anxious. On the contrary, connect with loved ones and build social networks. A single supportive friend can have a significant impact.

Social interaction can help you cope with life's ups and downs, provide support, and function as a distraction, all of which can be effective stress relievers.

Have extra time? To help others and yourself at the same time, consider volunteering for a charity.

4. Become Assertive.

Even if it would be nice to do everything, there is a cost involved. You may better control your to-do list and stress levels by developing the ability to say no and being willing to delegate. In the pursuit of well-being, healthy boundaries are crucial. Everybody has boundaries—both physical and emotional.

Accepting may appear like the simple solution to maintaining harmony, averting confrontations, and completing the task at hand. Instead, because your needs and your family's needs come second, it could lead to internal conflict in you. Anxiety wrath, anger, and even the impulse for revenge can arise from putting oneself last. And that's not a very composed and serene response. Recall that you come first.

5. Practice yoga.

Yoga is a well-liked method of reducing stress because of its sequence of poses and breathing techniques. Yoga combines mental and physical practices that could assist you in achieving body and mind harmony. You can reduce tension and anxiety by practicing yoga.

Take a class or try yoga on your own; classes are available everywhere. Particularly because of its softer poses and slower tempo, hatha yoga is an excellent way to release tension.

6. Get adequate rest.

You may have trouble falling asleep if you're anxious. Your sleep quality might be negatively impacted by having too much to accomplish and too much on your mind. However, sleep is when your body and mind regenerate.

Your attitude, energy level, ability to concentrate, and general functioning can all be impacted by how well and how long you sleep. Make sure you have a peaceful, calming bedtime ritual if you struggle with sleep. Consider keeping a routine, putting phones and iPads away, making sure your sleeping space is cold, dark, and silent, and listening to calming music.

7. Observe Journalling

Pent-up emotions can sometimes be released by writing down your thoughts and feelings. Allow it to happen without premeditating what to write. Jot down whatever that occurs to you. Nobody else has to read it. Therefore, don't try to use perfect syntax or spelling.

Write down your ideas or just put them on the computer screen. When you're done, you can either delete what you wrote or keep it for later consideration.

8. Be inventive and melodic.

Playing or listening to music might help you decompress. It can relieve mental strain, relax muscles, and lower stress hormones. Increase the volume and allow the song to completely engross you.

If you're not interested in music, focus on another pastime you like. Try sewing, gardening, reading, or drawing, for instance.

9. Discuss it.

Stress has the ability to turn molehills into mountains. Stress management can be particularly challenging when the brain is overloaded. Try discussing it with a close friend or even in front of the mirror. Opening up about unpleasant thoughts can aid in their proper processing by the brain.

10. Give your favorite things some time.

Hobbies can help people decompress, whether their stress stems from handling changes in their lives or from feeling overscheduled. One easy method to practice self-love and assist the body in reducing stress is to make time for your favorite activities.

If self-care techniques aren't helping you decompress or if you're finding it difficult to handle new pressures, you might want to consider therapy or counseling. Additionally, seeking therapy could be a wise move if you feel helpless or stuck. If you find yourself worrying a lot, unable to maintain daily schedules, or failing to fulfill obligations at work, home, or school, you might also want to consider counseling.

You can acquire new coping mechanisms and identify the roots of your stress with the assistance of licensed counselors or therapists.

CHAPTER 10

CONCLUSION

Brooke learned in her 50s that colorectal cancer was serious and something she could overcome with willpower, encouragement, and a renewed sense of purpose. Even the healthiest among us occasionally need to pay attention to the whispers of life's unforeseen obstacles, as she reminded her community while tending to her garden.

Collins decided to devote his life to raising awareness of colorectal cancer after being moved by his personal experience and the comfort that comes with early detection. He worked as a volunteer for neighborhood cancer organizations, telling his experience at schools and community gatherings and inspiring others to take ownership of their health and face their family history.

Collins' commitment to doing frequent screenings has paid off over time. It not only helped him maintain good health but also gave his family a ray of hope and resiliency. With the knowledge that early detection and care could change their futures, the genetic legacy of colorectal cancer no longer appeared insurmountable.

Collins' tale came to represent an unshakable dedication to health and the effectiveness of early detection and prevention. He was a living illustration of how treating colorectal cancer seriously may make a huge difference, even in the face of inherited risk. Mark transformed into a health defender, paving the path for a better, cancer-free future in a family that had previously been plagued by the illness.

Colorectal cancer is not a death sentence. It is not a judgment imposed upon you. Although it is a struggle, we can rise to it together. You have learned the value of prevention and the strength of early detection throughout the duration of these pages. You now know that taking action can be the best way to combat this illness and that knowledge is your most powerful tool.

You can significantly lower your chance of developing colorectal cancer by making informed decisions. You can achieve regular screenings, stress management, exercise, and a nutritious diet. You are the creator of your future and the defender of your health. In this fight, your friends and family are your allies.

As you put this book away, keep in mind that prevention requires a lifetime of dedication. Remain compliant with screenings, lead a healthy lifestyle, and promote awareness among those in your social groups. Give what you've learned to others; knowledge truly is power.

Though our journey together comes to an end here on these pages, your path to a cancer-free, healthier future is only getting started. Face this problem with confidence, knowing that you have the means and expertise to safeguard your loved ones and yourself. Assume responsibility for your well-being, and let's collaborate to create a future in which colorectal cancer is a thing of the past.

Your commitment to prevention is a ray of optimism and a guarantee of better, healthier times to come.

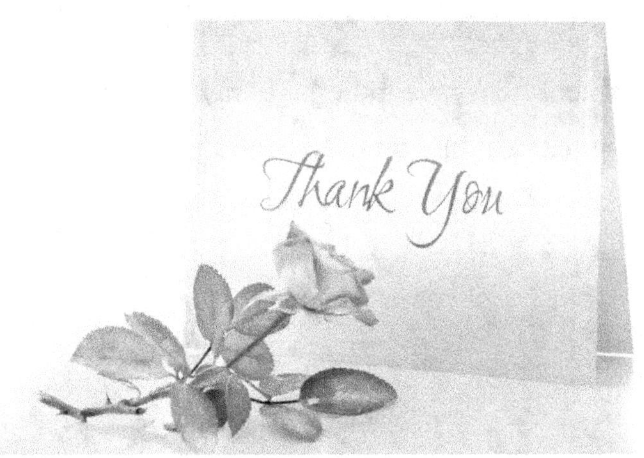
Thank You

www.ingramcontent.com/pod-product-compliance
Lightning Source LLC
Chambersburg PA
CBHW070819260726
48660CB00005B/1917